Health Unplugged

AuthorHouse™
1663 Liberty Drive
Bloomington, IN 47403

First published by AuthorHouse 7/20/2010

ISBN: 978-1-4520-2527-8 (sc)
ISBN: 978-1-4520-2528-5 (e)

Library of Congress Control Number: 2010908632

Printed in the United States of America
Bloomington, Indiana

This book is printed on acid-free paper.

Health Unplugged

James A. Robinson

Message

No one plans to fail
They just fail to plan!

Contents

Power of Choice

We control our own lives. What we want in our lives we can have, but we have to be clear and focused on what we want. In order for us to stay focused and clear with goals in life, we must be willing to give up something. God gives us everything that we need on this earth, but it's up to us to go out and create the world that we want. If you think you can do something, you will do it. If you think that you can't do something, you won't do it. You have to take some type of action in order for things to happen.

If you think you can go to college, focus on it, study hard, get good grades, and you will make it to college. If you want to be a bum and get up in the morning thinking you'll be happy living in a homeless shelter, begging for money, digging in the garbage, without thinking about how to better your life, you will be a bum. If you think about and focus on being a drug dealer and wake up in the morning thinking about selling drugs or buying drugs, you will get everything that comes with it (jail, death). It is important what you think and what your feelings are because it will show up in your life, good or bad. I think of positive thoughts, whatever the situation is, good or bad. I think about how to better myself through educating myself and helping others. I believed that I could finish high school, and I did. I believed that I could finish college, and I did. I believed that I could lose weight, and I did. But in every siutation, I had to give up time and money. It is important to have positive people around you because the job of negative people is to stop you from reaching your goals. When you get up in the morning, you have to put on a helmet, (like a football helmet) to deflect off the negative people around you (your lover, friends, family, and co-workers). You have to believe that you can lose weight in order for it to happen, but you have to give up time. You have to be willing to exercise at least 2-3 times a week. You have to give up money (healthy foods cost more money). You have to have a plan or goal, and this book will help you to achieve your goals.

I Can't Afford It

Negative people always say words like "I can't afford it" or "It cost too much," but what they are really saying is "I don't want to do it." A person will always manage to find money for whatever they want to do. Their motto is "Buy what I want and beg for what I need." Negative people, if you let them, can drain you mentally as well as physically. Relationships can be positive as well as negative. When you spend time around a positive or negative person, you adopt some of their traits, whether its directly or indirectly. If your husband or wife says, "Lets go to McDonalds, to eat" chances are you are going to eat what he or she eats. The thinking power of one affects the other. In a relationship you push, pull and vibe off each other's actions and thoughts. In a home, no one buys two sets of groceries. Everyone eats the same thing. If one person brings in fast food everyday that's what the household eats. Food and activities in a relationship are shared, not divided. To lose weight, you have to think as an individual. Your partner may not want to eat healthy food, but for you to lose weight, you have to think about yourself. If your partner really loves you, he or she will see that you are trying to doing something positive with your life and relationship.

So, if you tell your partner to stop bringing fast foods and sodas in the house but your partner doesn't stop, you have to take it upon yourself to buy food for your home to make it healthy. You have to exercise or go to the gym when he or she is lying in the bed tired. In the end, whether you choose to gain or lose weight, it all falls upon you. You cannot depend on someone else to make decisions about your health or lifesyle. Friends, family and co-workers can be your biggest supporters or worst enemies if they don't understand what you are trying to achieve. It's all about you. Watch out for words like, "Man, you are fat", and "You need to lose weight." When you lose weight, watch out for words like, "Man, you lost a lot of weight," or "You don't need to lose anymore." People will always try to distract you from accomplishing your goals. Remember, that is the job of a negative person.

Kitchen 101

The dominant person in the relationship will generally determine the types of food brought into the home. If there are children in the home, they will mimic what their parents do and adopt the same eating habits. First, the kitchen, the cabinets and the refrigerator have to be reconstructed. You have to rid them of all white stuff! White bread, flour, noodles, spaghetti, rice, etc. Also get rid of gallons of whole milk, half gallons of juice, liters of sodas, large bags of cookies and candy. If you have these products in your home, when they are finished, do not buy them again. Sweets like cookies and candy should be bought in single portions, do not buy them in gallons and big bags. Do not buy liters of sodas and store them in your home, because if it is there, you will eat it or drink it. Buy your cookies and candy in indivual servings, and buy milk in either a pint or a quart. When that is all gone you will not feel the need to run out to the store in the middle of the night because you will have satisfied your craving.

The Lost Art

A friend of mine at work told me he spends at least $6 to $8 a day on lunch and wanted to start bringing food from home instead. His reason for not bringing his food was because he didn't have the time to prepare it. He was gaining weight from eating fast food for lunch everyday. I told him that time is the key to losing weight and that cooking your food has become a lost art. When I was a kid, I didn't see a McDonalds, or any fast food restaurant until I was about 20 years old hanging out with my friends and chasing girls. Over the years I gained about sixty pounds, but I lost it in over 8 months. You have to start eating slow foods, not fast foods. Everybody wants everything fast, right away. Just consider the microwave, Jenny Craig and Nutri-System, you just pop your food in and its ready in a second. That stuff doesn't work. It costs too much, and after a while you get tired of the same foods. Cooking your own food is the best way to losing weight and to keeping it off. That means breakfast, lunch and dinner. Buying and cooking your own food makes you the boss of your diet, not some teenage kid deep frying in the back of a fast food or chain restaurants. I know that you have heard about the nasty things that they do to your food in those places, like putting fries in their noses, spitting in food, dropping your food on the floor, taking bathes in the sink and so on. I don't know about you, but it scares me. Americans are so lazy and we are the fattest people in the world. Do you know how people from other countries recognize Americans? They just pick out the fat ones!

There are some foods and chemicals I had to learn about before I could lose weight and keep it off. I also had to learn about conventional foods ,organic foods and portion size. We as Americans and some Europeans, don't eat food, we eat fast foods. My friends always say , "I don't have time to cook". But 60 years ago, before fast food , people found time to cook. Educating yourself about food is the key.

Wheat Treat

Wheat, in it's natural unrefined state, has a lot of good nutrients. To get the benefits of these good nutrients, it is important to choose whole wheat products from whole wheat flour rather than products with refined flour. Refined flour removes most of the nutrients from wheat. There are two big differences between white and wheat : how they are processed and how healthy they are. The flour of both is made from wheat berries, which have three nutrient-rich parts: the bran(the outer layers), the germs(the innermost area), and the endosperm(the starchy part in between). Whole wheat is processed to include all three nutrutious parts, but white flour uses only the endosperm. White flour is dead bread. Flour used to make white bread is chemically bleached , just like your clothes. So, when your are eating whitebread, you are also eating chemical bleach. Whole wheat is much higher in fiber, vitamins B and E, magnesium, zinc, folic acid and chromium. Try brown rice, whole wheat noodles, wheat bread and bran cereals.

Fiber

Fiber is the only substance we eat that does not digest. This means fiber has no calories. When you eat food rich in fiber, it gives you a sense of fullness. When you are full, you eat a lot less. Fiber can be found in fruits, vegetables, whole-grain breads, cereals,and starchy vegetables like potatoes, but not potato chips or french fries. If you are trying to lose weight, cutting out your fiber would be crazy. Not only does fiber fill you up without making you fat, it is also beneficial to your overall health. It helps with your digestion and helps to keep you regular. Fiber contributes to the overall well-being of the digestive track and helps to reduce risks of diseases, such as heart disease and certain cancers. Meat, white flour products (bagels, white bread, white bread crackers and most muffins), candy, soda and all sweets can be an issue because they don't contain fiber.

Your Metabolism

What factors determine your metabolic rate? Your metabolic rate is the amount of calories your body uses every day. The basal metabolic rate (BMR) is the rate your body uses energy for vital body processes. The rate you burn energy during physical activity and the rate you use energy during digestion of food are the two other factors involved in your total metabolic rate. To improve your metabolic efficiency all you need to do is alter what you eat and what you do a little bit, in order to experience a difference in how you look and feel. The best way to jump-start your metabolism is to exercise. Exercise will reduce body fat and increase lean muscle mass. By increasing your lean muscle mass, your metabolism will increase and aid in the weight-loss process. Muscle tissue uses more calories than fat tissue because muscle tissue has a higher metabolic rate. Aerobic exercise, like walking, swimming or cycling, has the added bonus of speeding up your metabolism for 4 to 8 hours after you stop exercising. Additional calories will be burned off long after you stop exercising.

Breakfast is Essential

If your body has been deprived of food throughout the night, your metabolism has slowed down. If the cells do not receive sufficient nutrients they will begin to function less efficiently on smaller amounts and they will actually store more fat to use during these times of nutritional deprivation. Eat 4 small meals a day to keep your body's fuel supply consistent and to keep your metabolism revved up. Avoid eating late at night. Your metabolism naturally slows down in the afternoon and evening, so eat a hearty breakfast. Consistency is important because your body's metabolism adapts to your current weight. If you have been dieting or skipping meals, your body's metabolism slows down to compensate for the lack of nutrients. When lean people overeat their metabolism speeds up and when obese people diet, their metabolism slows down. The key is a balance of exercise and diet.

Eat fewer High-Fat Foods and Less Total Calories

Choosing healthy foods, such as lean protein and vegetables, can actually increase your metabolism as well. You should increase your dietary fiber, limit sugary foods, alcohol and caffeine and don't smoke. The best foods to increase your metabolism and help you lose weight are fish, dark green leafy vegetables, tomatoes, blueberries and other fruits, whole grains and at least 8 glasses of water a day.

Weight Lifting, Resistance, and Strength Training

Weight lifting and training do not speed up your metabolism. They burn fat and increase your lean muscle mass, which increases your resting metabolic rate. A combination of aerobic exercise and resistance training is best for optimal fat burning and metabolism boosting. If you exercise in the morning, you will reap the benefits of a faster metabolism throughout the day. Exercise in short 10 or 15-minute bursts every couple of hours to keep your metabolism pumping. Exercise any time you can fit it into your day and you will burn that fat away. By exercising just a little more than usual, you can speed up your metabolism and use up stored fat in the process.

Halt on Salt

Table salt is another name for sodium chloride. Sodium is found in a lot of foods. We do need salt in our diets, but it is not good to overdo it. When watching your weight, you should also be careful of water weight which occurs due to your salt intake. The more the food is processed the more salt it contains. You can find sodium in: table salt, baking soda, soy sauce, horseradish, MSG, pickles, sauerkraut, processed meats and cheeses, frozen dinners, salted chips, nuts, pretzels and canned soups. Foods that are labeled as cured, pickled, corned, or smoked are high in sodium. The less processed a food is, the lower the amount of sodium it has. Try to eat fresh or frozen instead of canned vegetables. Limit your processed food intake, and keep the salt in the cabinet instead of on the table. You should flavor your food with spices and herbs. Try not to use too many condiments: such as mustard, ketchup and soy sauce on your foods, it can add up. Here are the cold hard facts. The body requires only 500 milligrams of sodium each day. The American Heart Association recommends no more than 2,400 milligrams of sodium per day, but most of us take in more than 4,000 milligrams every day.

The Soda Blues

The way I look at it, soda and diet soda have only one good quality, which is they contain water. But the water is carbonated, so it is no longer really a good thing. If you want to feel good and look good, you need to put things in your body that it needs. Soda is full of artificial ingredients that the body must work to process. Anytime you give your body unnecessary things to process you keep it from functioning at an optimal level. Soda gives you artificial colorings, flavorings, and sweeteners to deal with, like high fructose corn syrup and aspartame. These items have no nutritional or health benefits. I quit drinking soda and diet soda, and I have to say I feel much better! Now that my soda addiction is gone, it's so easy to ignore, and now I crave water the way I used to crave sodas.

Drink filtered water. Watch out for water with salt and chemicals added for flavor. Did you know that Dasani water is filtered from tap water and was banned in the UK because its levels of bromine may cause cancer? Make your own juice with a juicer or blender, and make hot tea, Ice tea, or lemonade. And if you want vitamin water, just take a vitamin with your water! Can you guess which sodas have the highest calories and sugar?

In 1 can of Pepsi - 160 calories - 10 teaspoons of sugar
In 1 can of Coke - 159 calories - 9.5 teaspoons of sugar
In 1 can of 7-Up - 149 calories - 9 teaspoons of sugar
But the winner is ... Mountain Dew with 179 calories and 12.5 teaspoons of sugar! Studies show that sodas and diet sodas may cause obesity.

Glorified Tap Water

Companies like Coca-Cola and PepsiCo, with their Dasani and Aquafina bottled water products, spend millions of dollars on ads that depict freshness and purity... when in fact both of these brands, like many leading brands, use municipally treated tap water as the source. It is unrealistic to think that water can be bottled in plastic containers, produced at a bottling factory, transported and stored at high temperatures for months at a time and be purer than what a basic home water filtration system can provide. It is impossible to get chemical free water from a plastic bottle. Basic home water filtration is more convenient, produces higher quality water, and costs a fraction of what bottled water costs. It is 10 times the quality, 1/10th the cost, and has no pollution! Bottled water causes over 60,000,000 plastic bottles to be produced, filled, transported, and disposed of every day in America. It is an environmental nightmare and it takes 3 times as much water to produce the bottle as it does to fill it! Use of fossil fuels and the related emissions from transporting dense, heavy containers of water throughout America make it even worse. Plastic takes over 300 years to degrade in nature. Plastic was invented 140 years ago, and it is all still here, piling up in our landfills, oceans and communities. Seldom is there a great environmental change we can make that offers better quality and, more convenience at 1/10th of the cost. Switching from bottled water to home water filtration does just that. Quality in-home water filtration is by far the best way to ensure healthy water for you and your family. A single home or office water filtration system can prevent thousands of plastic bottles per year from entering and damaging our environment.

(Bisphenol A) Commonly know as
BPA
Safer plastic: 1, 2, 4, 5
Plastic to avoid: 3, 6, 7

Polycarbonate #7 is often found in baby bottles or Sippy cups, so use glass. Check the bottom of the plastic containers to check safety.

Juicing

Juicing regularly, aids in keeping organs such as your heart, liver, and kidneys strong and healthy. Juice also helps prevent colon cancer and keeps the digestive system in tiptop shape. This is because juices are great suppliers of protein, vitamins, and minerals. Juicing also helps your immune system, promotes good-looking, healthy skin, and makes you look younger. Other health benefits of juicing include flushing out fat and lowering cholesterol naturally. This helps you lose weight. Studies show that there is a link between diet and disease. Studies also show that a key factor to good health is the nutrients found in fruits and vegetables. Juicing fruits and vegetables allows these nutrients to go straight to work for you because they enter the bloodstream within minutes after drinking. I believe the benefits of juicing will provide a nutritional supplement to your diet that will lead to a happier and healthier lifestyle.

Message

Clean your Colon
It's impossible for you
To eat perfectly
The rest of your life

Mystery Meat

Eat only organic meat and dairy products, like beef, chicken, turkey, milk, cheese, and all dairy products. Get certified organic if you can. Meats that are not organic are loaded with growth hormones and, antibiotics. The meat comes from animals feed, modified soy, corn, and other drugs. These items lead to obesity. It is fine to eat these products as long as they are organic certified, ideally grass fed, and have not been injected with growth hormone, antibiotics, or other drugs. By eating foods that are not organic certified, you are putting a lot of animal growth hormones, powerful animal antibiotics, and other animal drugs in your body. This will create hormonal imbalances in the body leading to weight gain, abnormal storing of fat, menstrual cycle problems, PMS, and depression.

Farm Raised Fish

Did you ever wonder why some fish you buy at a supermarket or restaurant are all the same size? They are all raised in large fish tanks or fish farms. Farm raised fish live in cesspools of poisonous water, fish waste, and urine. They are fed large amounts of drugs and chemicals to increase growth and production. Most of the fish are injected with chemical food dyes and are fed modified corn. The chemicals and poison found in these fish cause hormonal imbalances leading to weight gain and depression. Try to buy your fish from old school fish markets, like our mothers and fathers used to do when we were kids.

Addiction / Emotional Eaters

Many reasons cause people to eat. Some people eat because of emotions and some eat because of a addiction. Addiction eating is like a sickness, it's something you can't control. An addiction is a chemical dependency on something. It's something that we feel that we can't do without. Fast food restaurants are like local drug dealers. The food is laced with all kinds of chemicals and processed sugars to keep you coming back so that the big companies can keep making money off of you. Like a drug addict, your body craves these substances. There is a beautiful golden arch on just about every corner and every time you see one, you are drawn in. People like convenience. How convenient is it that you only have to remember numbers 1-9 and not even really think about what you want? It's really nicely packaged with a burger, fries and a soda, and you can super size it for a few pennies more. How cool is that? When you stop eating these foods, you feel cravings and go through withdrawals. These withdrawals cause you to over eat to try to fulfill that need. The whole country is on legal drugs and it is all FDA approved!

Emotional eaters eat because of certain situations or events that they are dealing with in life. When we are not able to deal with certain things, we turn to food for comfort. We look to ice cream (by the gallon), soda, and tons of sweets to ease the pain. This is just a bandage, and you are only creating a bigger problem. What is considered as causes for emotional eating are:

- ❖ Death of a loved one (mother, father, siblings, child,)
- ❖ Husband or wife cheating, divorce
- ❖ Loss of a job, staying at a job you dislike,not getting a promotion
- ❖ Sickness (high blood pressure, heart problems, cancer etc…)

Portions are The Key

You have to learn to portion out your food. Its a proven fact that we are tempted to eat what is put in front of us. This may cause a person to eat 30 to 50 percent more than what he or she would usually eat. We have a tendency to eat until we are full or until there is nothing left on the plate. In doing this, we pack on a lot of unnecessary calories. If you do this, the funny thing is, depending on what you are eating, fifteen minutes later you will be hungry again. It is important to eat foods high in fiber and low in calories. One bagel is like eating 5 slices of white bread. Try sliced wheat toast instead. Portion your food with your eyes. Check out www.foodloversfatloss.com for a real good break down on portions.

<u>Organic and Lean Beef /Pork/ Fish</u>
1-Palm –Men-4-6 oz Women- 3-5 0z
<u>Breads</u>
1-2 Slices whole wheat /whole grain
<u>Eggs</u>
Egg whites, eggs substitute
Men -2 Women – 1

<u>Potatoes/ Spaghetti /Rice</u>
1 fist 1cup
<u>Cereals</u>
Men 2/3cup Women 1/2 cup 1cup, 1% milk, Low
fat, 1 cup
Check the serving size on the box
Sweets, cakes, ice cream less than 300 calories per
day

It takes 20 minutes for the stomach to tell the brain that we're full. When we eat family style, it's too easy to keep refilling the plate. Often we end up eating too much, just because it's in front of us. Here's how to control portion sizes to lose weight.The recommended meat portion is the size of a deck of cards. Fill the rest of the plate with vegetables and the rice, potato or pasta. The largest portion on the plate should be the vegetable. Never add rice, potato or pasta together in one plate or meal. Never eat rice, potato, pasta every day.

Eating Before Parties and Family Gatherings

Let's say a family gathering happened on Saturday around 3 to 5 O'clock in the afternoon. You skip your meals all during the day to prepare for the event. By the time you reach where you are going, you are very hungry and you tend to over eat. If you eat ahead of time, you will already be satisfied, and whether the food is ready when you get there or not, you will still be full so that you only eat a small amount instead of over eating. Events, like movies, family gatherings, parties, Thanksgiving dinner, Christmas dinner, New Years dinner,can cause you to overeat if you are not prepared. It is best to eat ahead of time because you cannot control what is being served at these affairs.

Left Overs

We all tend to eat and buy in quantity. A cookie, a sandwich, an order of fries, a candy bar, ice cream, or a bag of chips are all purchased by size or quantity. Trying to save a dollar, no matter what we buy, we eat until it is all gone. Think about it, how often do you take a bite of something or a spoonful of something and put the rest of it away for later? You know what they say about chips, "You can't eat just one." And it's the same with everything else that we eat. Not too many people eat a half slice of pizza or drink a half of a soda and save the rest for later. We may say that is what we are going to do, but come on, how many of us actually do it? Think about the ad for Alka Seltzer after over eating a meal, "I can't believe I ate the whole thing!" But you did. We can all relate to not being able to stop eating until everything is gone. Its funny, because most people don't like to go places and have second servings of anything. They have a fear of looking greedy to others, but they don't have a problem with the words like, medium, large, extra large, and oh yeah don't forget my favorite, super size. In the end no matter how you count , it all adds up to the same results, and we always eat until it is all gone. When you order larger sizes, in order to spend less money, it will always add up to the same prices, extra calories and weight gain.

Types of Vegetarians

One thing that many people don't realize or understand is that there are different types of vegetarians. Each individual vegetarian has his or her own personal reasons for choosing their diet, and these reasons determine exactly what foods they eliminate. Below is just a brief definition of each type of vegetarian.

Vegetarians can be separated into four types:

Semi vegetarians - These vegetarians eat all types of foods in their diet, including meat. However these individuals limit the amount of animal products they consume.

Lacto vegetarian - Individuals in this group are a step up from the semi vegetarians. They avoid all animal products except for dairy products in their diet.

Lacto-ovo vegetarians - This type of vegetarian diet excludes all meat except dairy and eggs. Not too different from the previous type.

Vegans - These are the hard-core vegetarians who avoid all animal products in their diets, such as meats, fish, dairy products, and eggs. The vegan diet relies on lentils, beans and soy products. Many new vegetarians compensate for not eating meat by overindulging in high fat dairy products and desserts, so watch out for sweet cravings.

Benefits of Vegetarian Diet

There are many benefits of a vegetarian diet. Today's emphasis on meat-centered diets has been proven to contribute too many of our modern illnesses. Choosing to eliminate or limit the meat you eat can bring you many of the health benefits of a vegetarian diet.

The number one cause of death in the United States (and other countries whose citizens eat a lot of meat) is heart disease. The consumption of meat, eggs, and dairy products, which are the three largest sources of dietary cholesterol, contribute greatly to heart attacks and other heart and circulatory problems. The average vegetarian has about 1/4 the chance of having a heart attack as the average non-vegetarian. For pure vegans, the risk is even lower. They have less than 1/10th the chance of having a heart attack as do non-vegetarians. Clearly, one of the greatest benefits of vegetarian diet plans is the decreased likelihood of heart and circulatory problems.

The benefit of a vegetarian diet is that vegetarians tend to naturally consume higher amounts of fiber. Vegetables, fruit, and whole grains are all good sources of dietary fiber, which meat-eaters often don't get nearly enough of. A lack of fiber is another major cause of digestive problems, including diverticulitis and colon cancer. The health benefits of a vegetarian diet also include reducing your share of the suffering that human beings inflict on animals. The average American consumes 2,714 land animals during his or her lifetime. Many of these factory-farmed animals are raised under inhumane conditions. If you were to stop eating meat, or even cut back substantially, you could literally prevent the suffering and death of hundreds, if not thousands, of animals.

And, since cows produce vast amounts of methane (a large contributor to global warming), another benefit of a vegetarian diet would be a reduction in factory-farmed beef. Among the other benefits of vegetarian diets, is a reduction in the global cow population would benefit everyone for generations to come.

The Calorie Count Down

Men need approximately 2,100-2,500 calories per day and women need approximately 1,400-1,800 calories per day. Men need more calories per day because they have larger muscles.

If you eat Dunkin Donuts bagel's with cream cheese, you will have just consumed 500 calories. Now add a 16 ounce carton orange juice that has 120 calories. It's lunch time, so you go to Burger King and have a fish sandwich with tarter sauce and a medium fries, and that's 1,000 calories. Dinner time comes and no one wants to cook, so you go to Applebees and have a Fiesta Lime Chicken that has 1,280 calories. You have just taken in 2,900 calories for the day and that's not including your sodas, coffee, or tea.

Bagel with Cream cheese	500 (adds up to 5 slices of white bread)
Orange juice	120
Burger King	1,000
Applebees	<u>1,280</u>
Total	2,900

Breakfast

Buttermilk pancakes with maple syrup	890
Smoke sausage with scramble eggs	1,480

Lunch

McDonalds Grilled Chicken Club	570

Dinner

UNO Chicago Grill Deep Dish Pizza	<u>2,310</u>
Total	5,250

So, if you eat 5,250 calories per day subtract 2,500, and you are over your calories intake by 2,750 calories if you are a man and 3,450 if you are a woman. This is estimated at 1 pounds per week, which averages out to about 48 pounds a year.

Beer, Wine, Liquor (Calories)

Here are some calorie counts for 12 ounces of different beers:

Sierra Nevada Pale ale: 175	Michelob Ultra: 96	Sierra Nevada Pale Ale:175
Same Adams Lager: 160	Amstel Light: 95	Sierra Nevada Stout: 210
Pilsner Urquelli: 160	Miller Genuine Draft Light: 64	Stella Artois: 140
Michelob: 155	Anchor Steam: 153	Bud Light: 110
Guinness: 153	Bass Ale: 160	Guinness Stout: 153
Heineken: 150	Becks: 140	Budweiser Select: 99
Corona: 148	Budweiser: 140	Coors Light: 102
Budweiser: 145	Corona Light: 105	Miller Light: 96
MGD: 143	Guinness Draught: 126	

The average wine has about 275-300 calories per 12 ounces. Of course, one glass of wine isn't usually 12 ounces. You might drink half as much wine as you would beer, making wine slightly lower calorie.

Mixed drinks are about the same. Gin and tonic or vodka and cranberry have about 300 calories per 12 ounces. Margaritas are very bad: they have about 750 calories!

Message

*Juicing flushes out fat and
Lowers cholesterol naturally*

How to Read Labels

The first place to start when you look at the Nutrition Facts label is the serving size and the number of servings in the package. Serving sizes are standardized to make it easier to compare similar foods; they are provided in familiar units, such as cups or pieces, followed by the metric amount and the number of grams.

The size of the serving on the food package influences the number of calories and all the nutrient amounts listed on the top part of the label. Pay attention to the serving size, especially how many servings there are in the food package. Then ask yourself, How many servings am I consuming (1/2 serving, 1 serving, or more)? One serving of beans and rice equals one cup. If you ate the whole package, you ate two cups. That doubles the calories and other nutrient numbers.

Calories and Calories from Fat

Calories provide a measure of how much energy you get from a serving of food. Many Americans consume more calories than they need without meeting recommended intakes for a number of nutrients. The calorie section of the label can help you manage your weight (gain, lose, or maintain.) Remember: the number of servings you consume determines the number of calories you actually eat (your portion amount).

There are 250 calories in one serving of beans and rice. How many calories from fat are there in one serving? Answer: 110 calories, which means almost half the calories in a single serving, come from fat. What if you ate the whole package? Then, you consume two servings, or 500 calories, and 220 would come from fat. Eating too many calories per day is linked to being overweight and obesity.

The Nutrients

The nutrients listed first are the ones Americans generally eat in adequate amounts, or even too much. Limit these nutrients. Eating too much fat, saturated fat, tran's fat, cholesterol, or sodium may increase your risk of getting certain chronic diseases, like heart disease, some cancers, or high blood pressure.

Most Americans don't get enough dietary fiber, vitamin A, vitamin C, calcium, or iron in their diets. Get enough of these nutrients. Eating enough of these nutrients can improve your health and help reduce the risk of some diseases and conditions. For example, getting enough calcium may reduce the risk of osteoporosis, a condition that results in brittle bones at old age. Eating a diet high in dietary fiber promotes healthy bowel function. Additionally, a diet rich in fruits, vegetables, and grain products that contain dietary fiber, particularly soluble fiber and low in saturated fat and cholesterol, may reduce the risk of heart disease.

The "Daily Value" on the Nutrition Facts label refers to the footnote in the lower part of the nutrition label, which tells you "%DVs are based on a 2,000 calorie diet." This statement must be on all food labels. But the remaining information in the full footnote may not be on the package if the size of the label is too small. When the full footnote does appear, it will always be the same. It doesn't change from product to product because it shows recommended dietary advice for all Americans. It is not about a specific food product.

These are the Daily Values (DV) for each nutrient listed, and they are based on public health expert's advice. DVs are recommended levels of intakes. DVs in the footnote are based on a 2,000 or 2,500 calorie diet. Note how the DVs for some nutrients change, while others (cholesterol and sodium) remain the same for both calorie amounts.

Eat "Less Than"

The nutrients that have upper daily limits are listed first on the footnote of larger labels and on the example above. Upper limits means it is recommended that you stay below (eat less than) the Daily Value nutrient amounts listed per day. For example, the DV for Saturated fat is 20g. This amount is 100% DV for this nutrient. What is the goal or dietary advice? A person should eat less than 20 g or 100%DV for the day.

Eat "At Least"

The DV for dietary fiber is 25g, which is 100% DV. This means it is recommended that you eat at least this amount of dietary fiber per day.

The DV for Total Carbohydrate is 300g or 100%DV. This amount is recommended for a balanced daily diet that is based on 2,000 calories, but it can vary, depending on your daily intake of fat and protein.

The Percent Daily Value (%DV)

The % Daily Values (%DVs) is based on the Daily Value recommendations for key nutrients but only for a 2,000 calorie daily diet, not 2,500 calories. You, like most people, may not know how many calories you consume in a day. But you can still use the %DV as a frame of reference whether or not you consume more or less than 2,000 calories.

The DV also makes it easy for you to make comparisons. You can compare one product or brand to a similar product. Just make sure the serving sizes are similar, especially the weight (e.g. gram, milligram, ounces) of each product. It's easy to see which foods are higher or lower in nutrients because the serving sizes are generally consistent for similar types of foods, except in a few cases like cereals. Nutrient Content Claims: Use the DV to help you quickly distinguish one claim from another, such as reduced fat vs. light or nonfat. Just compare the DVs for Total Fat in each food product to see which one is higher or lower in that nutrient. This works when comparing all nutrient content claimless, light, low, free, more, high. Look at the DV for calcium on food packages so you know how much one serving contributes to the total amount you need per day. Remember, a food with 20%DV or more contributes a lot of calcium to your daily total, while one with 5%DV or less contributes a little.

Trans Fat: Experts could not provide a reference value for trans fat nor any other information the FDA believes is sufficient to establish a Daily Value or %DV. Scientific reports link trans fat (and saturated fat) with raising blood LDL (bad) cholesterol levels, both of which increase your risk of coronary heart disease, a leading cause of death in the US.

Protein: A DV is required to be listed if a claim is made for protein, such as high in protein. Otherwise, unless the food is meant for use by infants and children under 4 years old, none is needed. Current scientific evidence indicates that protein intake is not a public health concern for adults and children over 4 years of age

Sugars: No daily reference value has been established for sugars because no recommendations have been made for the total amount to eat in a day. Keep in mind; the sugars listed on the Nutrition Facts label include naturally occurring sugars (like those in fruit and milk) as well as those added to a food or drink. Check the ingredient list for specifics on added sugars.

Science Fiction

Some food labels contain unfamiliar ingreditients. Let's break it all down and see what we are really putting in our bodies. Check your labels on your sodas and foods, (I'll give you a minute). Time's up! Here are the answers:

High fructose corn syrup (Plain and simple) its modifed corn that's made in a lab and is substituted for sugar. It's cheaper for companies to make so that's why they put it in all the foods that we eat. (STOP!)

Go to your kitchen and you will see it in all the food that we eat and drink, from sodas and, ice cream to morning cereals. It is addictive and it causes obesity.

Aspartame-(Plain and Simple) is an artificial sweetener, and it is 180 times sweeter than sugar. This is mostly found in sodas and foods that have ZERO or no calories on the label(Diet or Fat Free). Have you ever wondered why soda is sweet with out sugar? It is called Aspartame, aka Equal, NutraSweet, and Canderel. Tests have shown that it can be addictive, but in small dosages it's not supposed to be harmful. Lab test have shown that Aspartame has caused cancers in mice and can cause brain cancer in humans.

Dextrose-is also a corn-derived caloric sweetener. Its modifed corn made in a lab and substituted for sugar. Like corn syrup, dextrose contributes to our habit of more than 200 calories of corn sweetener per day. This is mostly found in cookies, bread, and crackers. Just like all other sugars, dextrose is supposed to be safe if taken in moderate amounts.

Blue #1 and Blue #2-Blue purple and green foods such as beverages, cereals, candy and iceing contain dyes that have been linked to cancer in animals.

Yellow 5 and Yellow 6-A common food coloring found in puddings, bread mix, chips and cookies. These dyes have been linked to learning and concentration disorder in children.

GMOs

Companies like Monsanto have been selling the idea of super food crops like GMO corn, soy and wheat for years, yet concerns about health and environmental safety remain.

The United States and Canada consume genetically modified organisms (GMOs) in around 70% of the foods we buy in grocery stores. By comparison, consumers in the European Union nations, Japan, China, Australia, New Zealand and other countries are able to avoid GMOs because their governments require mandatory labeling on foods that contain genetically engineered ingredients.

According to Consumers Union, 95% of consumers in the U.S. want products containing genetically modified organisms to be labeled. Yet, in 1996 the FDA ruled that genetically modified foods were not substantially different from others and need not be labeled. The FDA ruled that it wouldn't require the labeling of genetically modified meat or fish. Genetically Modified Organisms ("GMOs") are present in almost every prepared food in supermarkets today. Unless the package says "organic" or "non-GMO," you can be reasonably sure that any soy, corn, or wheat in most commercial foods has been genetically modified.

For a food source that has become so common, it's almost shocking how little we actually know about the long-term safety implications – and how little the general public knows about GMO foods at all.

Check the stickers on the fruits we buy in the supermarket
 They have 4 numbers on the stickers like # 4040 or #9045
Numbers starting with # 3,4 conventionally grown,
with pesticides (it is not organic). #8 Frankenstein food
(GMO) genetically modified foods # 9 organically grown

The Benefits of Vitamins

We need vitamins to function properly. Each of the 13 essential vitamins (A, C, D, E, K, B12, and the 7 B-complex vitamins) provides the regulation of a crucial function. We acquire a majority of the vitamins our body needs from food. When there is a deficiency, we are in danger of becoming seriously ill or even dying. Vitamin supplementation can reverse illness caused by vitamin deficiency, sometimes miraculously. It is rare to find someone who isn't taking a daily multivitamin. Since there is a good chance that most of the individuals who take a daily multivitamin are eating a variety of foods, is it really necessary that they take a multivitamin? It may not be necessary, but everyone can benefit from taking a multivitamin.

The benefit of taking a multivitamin is to prevent deficiency. In some situations your dietary needs may increase. Pregnant women are generally advised to start taking multivitamins. This is to ensure that they receive the proper nutrition and pass it on to their unborn child. By taking a multivitamin every day, a pregnant woman can decrease her risk of passing malnutrition on to her baby.

Another benefit of taking multivitamins is that it combats stress. There are numerous stress formulations that can keep you mentally healthy as well as energize you. Taking a multivitamin every day can also reduce your risk of cardiovascular disease and cancer.

Yoga

The benefits of yoga practice goes far beyond the actual time you spend in the poses. One of the most common reasons why people begin practicing yoga is to improve health and well-being. Yoga means union. It is a union of the mind, body, and breath. All aspects of your life are impacted by your practice.

The stretching that you engage in during every practice helps lengthen and stretch muscles, which helps reduce the risk of injuries.

The majority of yoga practices include some type of balancing in the poses. A significant number of people, especially as they began to get older, start to have problems with balance, and this can lead to major injuries due to falls. By having a greater sense of balance, you are able to move more easily and safely.

Tense muscles often contribute to pain. Relaxing muscles helps to minimize muscle tension and the pain associated with it. Also, breathing deeply into muscles helps lessen pain by altering your perception of it.

Yoga works all the muscles in your body. It helps strengthen and tone them and also builds endurance and stamina.

Carrying tension in your body takes an enormous toll on your energy reserves. By learning how to relax through your yoga practice, you benefit by enjoying higher levels of energy so you can more thoroughly enjoy your daily activities.

Most people breathe high in their chests. This does not allow them to get sufficient oxygen and it also triggers the stress response, which contributes to feelings of anxiety. Breathing deeply as practiced in yoga, helps relax your muscles and brings much needed oxygen to your cells. The deep sense of relaxation also leads to better quality sleep.

Each yoga practice ends with some type of relaxation. Since your body and mind are one, by relaxing your body you also relax your mind. Many yoga experts believe that a relaxation pose is the most beneficial pose in any yoga practice.

During your practice, you are focusing your attention on your breath and turning inward. This concentration allows you to withdraw from the distractions in your environment. A significant benefit of yoga practice is that you can take this ability to focus your attention into every aspect of your life. You can be fully present with whatever you are doing instead of worrying about tomorrow or regretting yesterday. Not only will your actions be more productive, you will also enjoy them in a greater way.

Deep breathing helps reduce the hormones that are released when you are feeling overwhelmed, overloaded, and frazzled. The internal focus that accompanies the poses helps create a relaxation response in your body.

The Benefits of a Massage

The physical benefits of massage include reduction in muscular pain and discomfort. The unseen benefits are what many people seek as a natural therapy to counteract and defend against the symptoms of modern day living.

It is recognized that massage therapy is an accepted method in not just maintaining but also in improving the mind's performance and agility. By using facial and head massage, you should respond over time with positive results such as greater mental focus and, improved concentration, and, as a result you will be able to think more clearly. Regard it as similar to the benefits that are provided by regular quality deep sleeps.

A good massage can reduce a person's current level of stress. It is a fact that a sizeable portion of sufferers from stress look for and use short term solutions such as nicotine, alcohol, and medication, prescribed or otherwise. These may well provide a short term fix, but in reality they may do more harm than good. It requires a gradual change of behavior coupled with enjoying the mental benefits that massage can offer. Don't forget, there is also the distinct advantage of it being a natural remedy.

Massage is also known to provide relief from the curse of headaches. By using various massage types, the tension that has built up in pressure points can be relieved, and the patient feels inner calmness, when the inherent stress levels are reduced and replaced with the beneficial feeling of wellbeing. High blood pressure can also be addressed and successfully reduced.

Massage on a regular basis provides an overall improvement in the relaxation of the body and mind. And if a person is more relaxed, he or she will create the conditions to be more productive, happier, and have a better and more positive outlook in life. The need for the feeling of relaxation is so much more important in today's fast paced world.

Message

*Eat slowly. It takes the brain
15 to 20 minutes to register that you are
full*

What Foods to Substitute

Fast Foods = Slow Foods, cooking your own meals Breakfast, Lunch, Dinner

Fried Meats, Turkey, Chicken, Pork, Fish = Grilled or Baked in oven

Eggs = Eggs Substitute, Egg whites, Organic eggs, Vegetarian eggs

Sodas, Diet Soda, Carton Juice = a Juicer or Blender, apples, orange, grapes, and make your ice tea, hot tea and lemonade, with real cane sugar

Whole milk = Soy milk, 1% Organic milk, Non fat, Low fat milk

White bread = 100% Whole Wheat, Whole Grain

Pizza Hut, Domino Pizza = Whole Wheat Crust , Prego , 100% All Natural Sauce , 2% Cheese or Low fat cheese, 15 min in oven

Cheese = Low fat cheese, 2% Cheese, Veggie Cheese made with soy

White Spaghetti, Pasta = Whole Wheat Spaghetti, Pasta

Pancake Mix = Whole Wheat blend, Pancake & Waffle mix

Butter = Smart Balance Butter Omega -3, Low fat butter

Syrup = Low fat, Light syrup, Maple syrup

Jelly = Organic Jelly, All Natural Jelly

Oil = Extra Virgin Olive Oil, Smart Balance Oil with Omega-3

Ice Cream=Breyers, All Natural Ice Cream (1 pint only per week)

Cookies, Cakes, Pies 1 serving = under 300 cal, 1-2 slices per day

Liquor, Beer, Wines = 1-2 glass per night

Bottle \Tap Water = Brita Filter water or other filtered water

Teflon or Non stick pans = Stainless steel pans

Microwave = Toaster Oven

What to Eat

Remember, cooking your food is the key to losing weight. The calorie count in food from the supermarket is lower than the calorie count in fast food restaurant foods. So, if you don't have the time, to cook your food, make the time, breakfast, lunch, dinner. Eat organic food if you can. 100% organic means the foods has no manmade chemicals, preservatives, or drugs. Organic means the product is 80% organic. When the labels say, "Made with organic ingredients," it means 30% of the product is organic. All natural is ok, but you have to read the label to make sure there are no chemicals in the food. One of the biggest problems people seem to have about being on a weight loss diet is the selection of foods they are going to be allowed to eat, not to mention, the selection of foods they are no longer going to be allowed to eat. The big fear some people have is that they will get tired and or bored of eating the same healthy foods over and over again. Some people may even go as far as to say it's impossible to consistently eat the same few healthy foods every single day for a long period of time without falling off the diet.

I eat the same foods at the same time of the day every single week/month/year and have been doing so for years now. I realize how crazy that may sound to some people, but to me there's nothing wrong with it. It's very convenient and simple. I really like the foods I eat. I am perfectly happy with these foods. After all, that's why I made them a part of my diet in the first place. I am certainly not telling anyone to eat like this, and you certainly don't have to. I'm just saying some people don't need that much variety in their diet. If you are the type of person who does want variety in your weight loss diet because you would get tired of eating the same foods over and over again, this list is for you. The key to losing weight (or any weight loss diet for that matter) is total calories consumed. Weight loss happens when you are in a calorie deficit, meaning you are taking in fewer calories than your maintenance level and are therefore burning more calories than you consume. While the foods on this list would all make great additions to your diet (for both weight loss and all around health), you need to make sure you stay within your calorie range. Also try to stay close to the guidelines regarding how much protein, carbs and fat your diet should consist of.

Here's a list of acceptable and healthy diet foods:

Grocery list

Lean Cuts of Beef	Milk (1% or skim)	Grits
Lean Cuts of Pork	Cottage Cheese Low Fat	Goya Rice
Lean Cuts of Lamb	Yogurt (Low Fat/Nonfat)	Chili
Lean Cuts of Veal	100% Whole Wheat Bread	Split Pea Soup
Organic Eggs	Whole Wheat Bagel	Green Pea Soup
Egg Whites	Whole Wheat Pita	
Tuna Fish	Wheat/Whole Grain Pasta	Whole Wheat Rolls
Salmon	Sweet Potatoes	Whole Wheat Hamburger Buns
Shrimp	Yams	1 Serving Cookie
Lobster	Oatmeal	1 Serving Cake
Flounder	Bran Cereals	1 Serving Chips
Sardines	Cheerios	1 Serving Breyers Ice Cream
Swordfish	Brown Rice	Homemade Tea
Trout	Organic Vegetables	Homemade Lemonade
Snapper	Organic Fruits	100% Organic Juice
Crabs	All Nuts	
Scallops		

Vegetarian Food

Veggie Cheddar Cheese	Veggie Cheese	100 %Whole Wheat Bread
Veggie Beef Strips	Egg Substitute	Whole Wheat Spaghetti
Veggie Chicken Strips	1% Organic Milk	Whole Wheat Pasta
Veggie Chicken Nuggets	Organic Eggs	Whole Wheat Hot Dog Buns
Veggie Ribs	Vegetarian Eggs	Whole Wheat Rolls
Veggie Chicken Cutlet	1% American Cheese	Wheat Pancake Mix
Veggie Hot Dogs	Low-Fat Yogurt	Whole Wheat Biscuits
Veggie Lunch Meat	Sherbet	Brown Rice
Veggie Sausage	1% Milk	Bran Cereal
Veggie Burgers	Breyers Ice Cream 150 Cal 1 Serving	Whole Wheat Waffles
Veggie Chicken	1 Serving Cookie	Kashi Pizza
Veggie Bacon	1 Serving Chips	Kashi Products
Tofu	1 Serving Cake	Fiber 1 Cereals
Patties		Cheerios

My friends always say there is a lot of sugar in fruits , and I always say that I have never, met anyone who got fat eating fruits and veggies -never.

All Fruits	Vegetables	Misc.
Apples	Spinach	Low-Fat Mayonnaise
Avocado	Tomatoes	Mustard
Bananas	Corn	Organic Jelly
Berries	Carrots	Peanut Butter
Cherries	Greens	Ketchup
Grapes	Lettuce	Olive Oil
Kiwi	Onions	Vegetable Oil
Lemon Lime	Potatoes	Low-Fat Dressing
Melons	Squash	Vinegar
Oranges	Zucchini	Low-Fat Syrup
Peaches	Broccoli	Low-Fat Butter
Pears	Beets	All Nuts
Plums	Soybeans	Popcorn 1 Serving
Grapefruits	Kidney Beans	Veggie Beans
Strawberries	Sun Flower Seeds	Veggie Soup
Bananas	Pinto Beans	Organic Soups
		Cane Sugar
		Domino Cane Sugar

Purchase items with words like: light, nonfat, less, low fat, 1%. It will help you to lose weight. You can purchase vegetarian meats from these supermarkets: Pathmark, Foodtown, Fresh Farm (has the smallest selections of the vegetarian meats, eggs and cheese, you really have to look hard to find it). Whole Foods and Trader Joe's (has the widest selection of organic meats, poultry, and organic eggs). And if you're a meat eater, try to cut back, it will help your health.

Eat real sugar and, stay away from Equal, Nutrasweet, Canderel (aka Aspartame) and Splenda. Use real sugar like raw cane sugar. People always say fruits have a lot of sugar, but fruits have natural sugar which breaks down in your body naturally unlike processed sugar. Buy your fruits from local farmer's markets if you can, if not, the supermarket is still a good choice.

Message

Eat your meals 30 to 60 minutes
Before you workout

The work out

Setting goals is the way to achieve anything you want in life, whether it's going to college, getting a job, or losing weight.

1. Clean your colon. It is impossible for you to eat perfectly for the rest of your life, so it is necessary for you to clean your colon at least once to twice a year.
2. Drink one-half to one gallon of pure water daily, to keep the cells hydrated and to flush toxins from your body.
3. Eat a minimum of one (organic if possble) per day: apples, grapes, grapefruit etc...
4. Have salad with lunch and dinner (organic if possble).
5. Never skip meals. It slows down your metablism. Eat breakfast, lunch, and dinner .
6. Eat every 4 hours, 7am until 8 pm. Never eat after 8pm (only have fruit or veggies).
7. Alway try to eat all your meals while moving around, not at night or while laying in bed.
   Breakfast: 7am - Lunch 12:00-1:00pm- Snack 3:00pm (all sweets under 300cals) per day- Dinner before 8:00pm (if possible) .

8. Eat your meals 30 to 60 minutes before working out. (You need fuel to work out or you will feel sick).

9. You should finish eating dinner 1 to 2 hour before bed. At night you store fat.

10. Listen to stress reducing DVDs once a week.

11. Buy a calendar and put it on the wall where you work out. Mark off the days that you work out. Example: Mon, Tues, Wed or Mon, Wed, Sat. Then set a 30, 60 or 90 day time period to lose 10-60 pounds.

12. Workout 30 to 60 minutes per day 3 times per week:

   a) Monday workout with weights 5 to 25 pounds

   b) Wednesday cardio or 30 minute walks, treadmill

   c) Saturday pushups and sit ups

   The goal is to mix up your workout during the week.

13. Buy a digital scale (a good one, something from $25 - $65).

14. Getting on the scale is like checking your credit score nobody wants to look at it. But it is important for your weight lost and health.

15. Every morning, immediately after using the bathroom, you should weigh yourself and mark your weight on your workout calendar everyday. The morning gives you your true weight for the day.

16. You will lose 5 to 10 pounds fast, and then your body will plateau and the weight lost will stop. Then take 1 to 2 days off. Then shock your body back with your workout. Be aware that men burn fat faster then women. So ladies don't stop your workout because your man is losing weight faster then you are, the weight will come off . You have to mix up your workout, get diffrent workout DVDs ,go swimming,or biking, use the treadmill, lift weigths, go skating, running, hiking, or walking at lunch time at work. The mix will help you take the weight off.

Your diet and exercise go hand and hand, so if you workout you will lose weight. But if you don't stop eating fast foods and restaurant foods you will gain the weight back guaranteed .

Travel Guide

When making travel reservations make sure to call ahead to the hotel and ask for a room with a microwave, a small refrigerator, and a gym. This allows you to stick to your food and workout plan. One of the hardest task is traveling with your food. You need to buy a set of 4-6.5 food containers for the week or weekend. It is also a good way to portion out your food.

When I travel, in my car for the weekend or vacation, I have a GPS, a toaster oven, a hot stove and a pan, a scale and juicer in my trunk.

I shop at the local supermarket in that city for my food and with my GPS I can always find a local supermarket, Whole Food, or Trader Joe's.

Message

Never skip meals.
It slows down your metabolism

Action Plan

I Will Start

_____

_____

_____

_____

_____

_____

_____

_____

_____

_____

_____

_____

Action Plan

I Will Stop

_____

_____

_____

_____

_____

_____

_____

_____

_____

_____

_____

_____

Notes

Grocery List

Fruits and Vegetables List

_____

_____

_____

_____

_____

_____

_____

_____

_____

_____

_____

_____

_____

Why I wrote this book

I wrote this book because I watched my Father have a stroke and die of heart disease, because of his diet. Over the years I gained 75 pounds eating fast food and over eating. I could not sleep at night from acid reflux. My asthma got worse and I was always so tired. My doctor said that I was boarder line diabetic and that I need to lose weight. So I made the commitment to lose the weight. I was small years ago at 165 pounds, and then my weight went up to 260 pounds. Now I'm back down to 185 and I have kept it off for two years. I learned that 80% of my weight problem was my diet. Now my doctor says that my blood, urine, heart, and my weight are at a good level. Now I have a diploma in Health and Fitness from Penn Foster Career School and Certified by ACSM American College of Sports Medicine. This book is from all the research and studying that I did over the years. I hope that it can help you achieve your weight goals.

Acknowledgements

Over the years, I have learned and have been influenced by many people. I would like to thank, and give credit to the following people: To my father, for showing me how to be a man. My mother for her love and strength, To my wife Arquilla Joyner, for helping me every step of the way, To my friend, John Latkovich for his thoughts and ideas, and I would also like to take this time to thank my family and my friends.

Thanks

James A. Robinson

For more information about James Robinson and the products and services available at Life(is)Inc Workouts, Food Plans, and Personal Trainers please call (212)-283-5177 (917)-468-8050 or email life.is2010@gmail.com

www.ingramcontent.com/pod-product-compliance
Lightning Source LLC
Chambersburg PA
CBHW020339290526
45785CB00005B/2097